Breast Cancer
the notebook

Written by Julia Chiappetta

with Dr. Merrick I. Ross, M.D., F.A.C.S
Professor of Surgical Oncology
M. D. Anderson Cancer Center

Published by Gemini Media, Inc.
P.O. Box 738
Acworth, GA 30101

August 2006 1st Printing
1 2 3 4 5 6 7 8 9 10

Library of Congress Catalog #: applied for

ISBN-10: 0-9787475-0-X
ISBN-13: 978-0-9787475-0-3
Printed in the United States

COVER DESIGNER: YVONNE BOOGAERTS
DESIGNER: AMANDA PFEIFFER
EDITOR: MOIRA GALLIVAN
COVER PHOTO: BOB CAPAZZO
BIO PHOTO: PAUL MCALLISTER

To my parents Olimpia and Charles, my life is rich because of what you have given to me so freely.

My dear Dr. Merrick Ross, thank you for your unconditional heart to help women and for being my friend.

To my sister and brother, Charlene and Palmer, I love you with all my heart.

Dearest Vincent, Briana, Victoria, Kim and Jackson; you all light up my life.

To my grandmother Julia, thank you for your love and prayers.

And I thank you Jesus, for your healing touch!

ACKNOWLEDGMENTS

Thank you Mark Chyrywaty for helping me sort through a maze of information and being by my side during this journey. To Lynn & Tony Ambrose, who were visiting with me when I found out I had breast cancer, thanks for being my rocks to lean on. Thanks to Jacqueline Urso who flew to Houston to be with me for my surgery, Rick & Stacy Urso for welcoming me into their home to recuperate and thanks to Joe Urso for guidance. To Bessie Pennie & Marilyn Bynoe my angels at MD Anderson. To Ann DeAngelo for sharing her personal and medical expertise. Thanks to Pastor Paul & Allison at Calvary Chapel Norwalk, CT for prayers. Alex Skora my research buddy, and Tim Dumas for constant guidance and encouragement. Thank you Pietro, Maria, Clara, Paula and Pedro Bria. Special thanks to Pedro for designing my web site. Special thanks to Dr. Carine Klein who taught me how to self examine and for her love and friendship. Thank you Dr. Ian Rubins, Dr. Mark Anderson, Dr. Amen Ness, Dr. Edward Jacobsen, Dr. Peter Dean, Dr. Stuart Epstein, Dr. Ivan Weinstein, Dr. Michael McGlynn, Dr. J. Books Hoffman, Dr. Douglas Masi, Dr. William Haggerty, Dr. Eduardo Blanco and Dr. Thom Sonnenberg – some of the finest doctors I have known. Thank you Gina & Jeff Anderson, Dolores Deck, Isobel Curcio, Aunt Sally & Uncle Babe, Larry Deluca, Aunt Mary, Barbara Urso, Bobby Carlson, Joann & Joey Camiglio, Jan Bryn, Philippe Soussand, Ulla Hansen, Rony & Linda Schlapfer, Prescott & Elizabeth Bush, Barbara Herrott, Santa & Joe Girard, Anna & Richard Zannino, Jane & Joe Carriero, Bernice Carroll, Milo & Marion Fuscaldo, Elizabeth Masterson, Maria Sullivan & Bruce Gulick, Pat Fuscaldo, Michelle Sanders, Ed Baker, and Tina Hansen. Special thanks to my prayer warriors, Pastor Bob Coy, Wayne Huizenga Jr., Pastor Stephan Tchividjian, Pastor Don Dukes, Lee Armfield, Mark Osborne, Suzanne & David Falkenstrom, Luis Palau Ministry, Beverley Hibbert, David Tinocco, Julie Johnson,

Grace Faison, Randy Bernsen, Deep Faith Ministry, John Montalvo, Alia & Brian Morilly, and Mia Nistico. Thanks to Angie Pietro & Donna Tomassetti who took me into their home after hurricane Wilma trashed my apartment. Special thanks to Moira Gallivan my editor for her kind heart. To Yvonne Boogaerts my graphic designer, Brigitte Cutshall my publisher, Paul McAllister, Amanda Pfeiffer, and dear Bob Capazzo thank you all for your expertise and kindness. Thanks to Lucille Perna & Harpo Curcio for their love throughout my life. From my heart I thank Nony Urso, Aunt Vivian, Aunt Conforte, Uncle Philip, Uncle Lindy and Uncle Romeo, you all touched my life in unique and profound ways.

INTRODUCTION
by Dr. Merrick I. Ross

Breast Cancer–the notebook is the result of the vision, dedication, hard work and generosity of an extraordinary woman, Julia Chiappetta. I first met Julia soon after her diagnosis and helped her through some difficult treatment decisions. I was further privileged to become her treating surgeon and have followed her carefully over the years and witnessed her ability to carry on with courage, optimism, vitality and empowerment.

At the outset of diagnosis, Julia spent long hours seeking information and treatment options while trying to grasp the complicated medical language necessary to understanding this disease. I helped her sort through these issues so she could come to a decision that she was comfortable with. I think Julia found the process very frustrating – she couldn't find a comprehensive resource that could address her issues and questions in a human way.

After her surgery, Julia had an epiphany that soon became her mission. Why not create a resource for newly diagnosed women with breast cancer that is easy to read and provides simple, relevant and accurate explanations? Although she asked me for assistance in making sure all information was medically correct, the idea, scope, intent and content is all Julia. I see it as a wonderful reflection of her persona.

Breast Cancer–the notebook is not only intended for you, the diagnosed, but also for your significant other, family and support team. Information available in this unique resource will be very useful to loved ones in helping you through this frightening and often confusing experience.

Since you may have more than one option for treatment, finding a physician who will spend time with you and your loved ones to sort through relevant issues and make clear confusing ones is important.

You need to feel that your treating physicians are part of your support team. You need to count on them to be open-minded but also compassionately straightforward in helping you come to a comfortable place about your treatment and the future.

Breast Cancer–the notebook, by design, is Julia's gift to you and your loved ones, providing guidance along your journey to recovery as well as helpful health maintenance strategies to improve your quality of life —during — and after — breast cancer. I feel privileged to have helped Julia, in my own small way, with this amazing endeavor.

FOREWORD
by Lynn Ambrose

I have had many close friends and relatives who have been diagnosed with breast cancer. All have taken different paths but only two have survived and are healthy and cancer-free today.

My role has been more of a sounding board and support system for each of these special women. Because of these women and after sharing their fight with them, I look at life with a greater awareness and I truly believe that we all need to stop and smell the roses and "enjoy the treasures of each day".

Julia (I call her Jules) has been a life-long friend of mine. We met in kindergarten and grew up in the same neighborhood. Our fathers knew each other and our grandfathers were the best of friends (they were deceased before either of us was born). It was inevitable that Jules and I would become eternal friends. We had so many things in common. We were born 12 weeks apart (she is older than me) and are both first born children. There have never been any secrets between us and yet our personalities could not be more different. Jules and I "just clicked" and we were referred to as the "groovy chicks" growing up.

Jules was the last person on earth that I would have expected to be diagnosed with cancer. She is the most fit (inside and out) person I know. Julia is an avid runner and vegan, and is very spiritual. Her faith is so important to her that I feel it is the most significant factor as to how she lives her life.

I remember the night that Jules told me that she had been diagnosed with breast cancer. My husband and I had just moved in with Jules for a month while we were in between houses. We were finally moving back to the town we all grew up in after a 20-year hiatus. Jules supported the move back to town and played a big role in making it come together. I remember my first reaction when I heard her words — there must be a mistake — it wasn't possible. Then an awful feeling came over me, the same feeling of dread I had felt in the past so many times before. How could this be happening to another important woman in my life? Why is it always my closest friends and the women who take care of themselves? I quickly assured Jules that we were in this together and I would be by her side every step of the way. We would fight this dreadful invader and she would indeed win the battle. There was no doubt in my mind that Jules would find her own way to attack and I would be her 1st Lieutenant. That said, I would be lying if I claimed it was easy. It wasn't easy for any of us, especially Jules, but she never complained.

You will hear about Julia's long journey. It is very heart warming and yet painful, but, it is a journey that only Jules could have made. Jules has spent thousands of hours on research and in the end she fought her illness in a way that was true to who she is as a person and in her own way. Watching Jules in her struggle with breast cancer inspired me to better appreciate every aspect of my life.

I'm happy to say, our bond is even closer today from going through this eye-opening experience together. I look forward to each and every celebration with Jules (we celebrate a lot). I am thrilled that she has decided to share her story. I know it will change your life, as it has mine, and give you the strength to live each day in your own way.

FOREWORD
by Mark Chyrywaty

If we are fortunate, we can touch another person's life and help improve that person. If we are extremely fortunate, we can help them while they heal.

Before her diagnosis, I considered Julia to be one of the healthiest people I knew; she was full of energy, in excellent physical shape, ate well, and had exercised her entire life. When Julia first told me that she had breast cancer, it really shook me. I remember how hard it was for Julia to find the words to tell me she had cancer. She was terribly upset, she felt uneasy, uncertain and frightened. Julia was afraid of the unknowns — how much cancer was in her body, how fast it was spreading and what damage had already been done.

Too often, when we become ill, we isolate ourselves from others (afraid of exposing a perceived weakness). We need instead to find strength and reach out to others. Though it was difficult, Julia called her friends and family and shared the news of her cancer. She surrounded herself with positive, supportive and caring people. I encourage you to take this step of strength.

Our outlook determines our outcome. Healing begins with our attitude, and we decide it every day. The choice is ours. We can wrongly choose the attitude of a victim; thinking "there is nothing I can do" or "what did I do to deserve this"? This attitude brings greater fear, frustration, anger and depression. Or we can choose a better path, choosing to have an attitude of hope. With this thinking, we can face our fear and learn to overcome it. Julia showed great courage in facing her fears. She decided to fight and take action toward healing.

The full page of people Julia gives thanks to reveals that Julia did not go through her journey alone. Looking back, I see how each person took part during that period in Julia's life; she had the support of a wonderful family, compassionate church friends and exceptional physicians.

I believe my role was that of a friend and also as Julia's health counselor. We worked together and developed her personal plan for healing. Julia was searching for answers, and I shared with her all that I had learned about health. I had studied nutrition over the years, I read health journals and researched the functions of the body; I was completely fascinated with the way it works. I showed her that our bodies were designed to maintain balance, strengthen the immune system, fight off illness and keep us healthy. The body actually heals itself. Each cell is self-repairing, and each cell performs its job to keep our entire system healthy. But we control what goes into the body and what it is exposed to. Our responsibility is to provide the body what it requires to perform the necessary functions to stay healthy. If we nourish the cells, the body will respond.

To overcome the cancer, we wanted to understand what was preventing her body from containing and eliminating the cancer cells. One important step we took was to ask what stresses she had in her life: physical, chemical, environmental, and emotional. We assessed these stresses and figured out a plan to remove or reduce them. It was a matter of doing less of those things that were harmful and more of the things that were beneficial. I reminded Julia that the body is slow but efficient; she needed to be patient, stay focused, remain positive and never lose hope.

In order to fight cancer there are lifestyle changes to be made, and we need to know what and how much to change. We need information before we can take action. When we have reliable information we are able to make prudent decisions. Julia worked hard to learn about her body's needs and then changed her lifestyle. She changed her diet dramatically; she nourished her body with the foods it needed to heal itself. She changed her workouts, adjusting to moderate aerobics, moving away from stressful and taxing activities. She deepened her faith and relationship with our Lord, learning to trust and be comforted in difficult times. Julia changed and improved, she developed, and she grew healthy. This notebook is organized with information to help you make these important decisions.

It was wonderful to be a witness to Julia's strengthening, recovery, and transformation into an improved person on all levels. I am grateful that Julia has developed this notebook to help others with breast cancer. My hope is that this resource helps you in your healing.

May the Lord bless and heal you,

Mark J. Chyrywaty
Psalm 103: 2,3

YOU HEAR THE WORDS . . .

Breast Cancer

WHAT SHOULD YOU DO NEXT?

KNOWLEDGE IS POWER . . . . . .

but where do you start?

The word Cancer carries with it so many emotions
and you need help.

You are not a doctor and you do not have the time
to do research.

You are feeling alone, angry, afraid, confused
and panicked . . .

Help!

My hope is that this notebook provides a foundation of knowledge to help you on your own personal path towards living a healthy, positive and cancer-free life.

Oncologists (cancer doctors) wrote most of the books I read. Whilst I appreciated their efforts to provide information, the medical jargon slowed down my learning process and I would often need to stop and highlight words that were foreign to me and then research their meaning. I was able to glean some good information from each book I read, video I watched, website I researched, but much of it was repetitive, and did not meet my immediate needs. It was a tedious job, combing the wisdom of numerous sources, but I continued relentlessly—with an unquenchable thirst for knowledge.

This notebook is a synopsis of that research; a foundation of facts placed at your fingertips if you have just heard the painful words "you have breast cancer" or if you simply want some good information to take a preventative approach.

With a diagnosis of breast cancer, **we need information and we need it fast**...so, take a deep breath, dig in, do your homework and remember that *nothing* is impossible. You will get there by taking one step at a time. **Never doubt that you have the ability to do this!**

I am blessed to be healthy at this time, never forgetting that each day is a wonderful opportunity to live, share, laugh and have fun. My heart is to share with you what I have learned. I encourage you to begin making changes to do the things you can do right now, today, to get started.

The notebook is a gift from me to you to help and guide you. My heart and prayers are with you!

Be encouraged,

Julia

TABLE OF CONTENTS

I was the **one** in the **"one in eight"** women you hear about in the statistics. It was not someone on television, in the news, a neighbor nor a colleague.

IT WAS ME!

This is where I was when I began my own journey with breast cancer in March of 2000. I had some wonderful doctors who had cared for me most of my life, and the hospital in my hometown still smelled of fresh paint from a recent expansion and renovation. My family, friends, and church were all supportive of me, but it was still my responsibility to make the decisions necessary to take charge of my own body and health.

I had been working in the travel industry meeting the demands of busy clients, producing meetings and events so attention to detail and problem solving are strengths. I am also a strong believer in the power of prayer. I knew that I could best find my way if I could just amass and organize all the facts and get on my knees. After all, I live and breathe the credo "exhaust all possibilities". I am someone who never gives up hope; in my world the glass is not only half full, but over-flowing most of the time.

I began by ordering a multitude of videos and books, subscribing to newsletters offered by cancer web sites and doing hours of daily research on breast cancer and nutrition. One day early in this project, I glanced up from my computer screen to find a glorious spring day taking place outside my window. I briefly relaxed in the moment and then had an epiphany: I had a marathon of work ahead of me and race day was quickly approaching.

I had to devise a plan to win this race!

Life & Health = Commitment = Knowledge + Prayer

There are 10 trillion cells in our body. We function as living organisms because these cells work well together. Growing and dividing are their most basic function. Cells are the smallest parts of our body that are complete and living units. They divide to form more cells exactly like themselves, to repair damaged cells, and to replace old cells.

Like other cancers, breast cancer starts with a single cell. In the breast, that single cell is usually inside the lobules and ducts where lots of cells normally divide during part of the menstrual cycle. There are rarely symptoms of early breast cancer. The most common sign is a painless lump or thickening that does not go away or change with the menstrual cycle. Although breast cancer can occur anywhere in the breast, the upper outer quadrant is most commonly affected because 80% of breast tissue is located in this area.

• Lobules — spherical-shaped sacs in the breast that produce milk.

• Ducts — pathways in the breast where the milk passes from the lobules to the nipple; they are lined by cells that can become cancer.

• Lymph Vessels — a clear liquid consisting of white blood cells, proteins, and fat flow through these channels to the lymph nodes.

• Lymph nodes (also called lymph glands) — destroy and filter out bacteria before it passes to the bloodstream. Your body has many lymph nodes, mainly in the neck, armpit and groin and this system is a major route by which cancer spreads.

• Axilla — area under the arm where most lymph nodes drain from the breast

Each month, breast cells are signaled by way of the hormones estrogen and progesterone to begin dividing rapidly. This prepares the breast for pregnancy, ultimately for breast-feeding and the breast swell. If pregnancy does not occur, a second signal is sent for the breast cells to stop multiplying and the breasts shrink.

Every month and year this cycle of rapid cell growth inside the breasts is repeated. This raises the odds for abnormal cells to form and multiply. When that happens, millions of these cells have grown in one place and they form a tumor or lump.

The difference between healthy cells and cancerous cells is that the cancer cells don't care what the body needs. They won't stop when the body tells them to stop and they take on a life of their own.

When a cell becomes cancerous, several events take place, all involving its DNA. DNA is the blueprint inside every cell, in every plant and animal on earth. It carries codes that determine every feature in our bodies and is the link with our family. DNA is terrific, but it isn't perfect. It can be damaged, and sometimes that damage results in cancer.

Breast cancer occurs when cells in the breast grow out of control and invade breast tissue. It can spread to the lymph nodes as well as throughout the body.

These out-of-control cells form to become a tumor. Tumors that cannot spread are called benign tumors and tumors that are cancerous are called malignant tumors. It may take months or years for a tumor to form or to be large enough to feel.

Like a stealth terrorist, breast cancer usually grows silently and without any pain.

- The breasts of an adult woman are milk-producing, tear-shaped glands.

- They are supported by and attached to the front of the chest wall on either side of the breastbone or sternum by ligaments.

- They rest on the major chest muscle which is called the pectoralis major.

- The breast has no muscle tissue.

- A layer of fat surrounds the glands and extends throughout the breast.

- Each breast contains 15-20 lobules.

- The breast is mostly fat which helps to give it its size and shape.

- At the ends of the lobules are tiny glands or sacs where milk is produced if signaled by hormones.

- The areola is the darker pigmented area around the nipple.

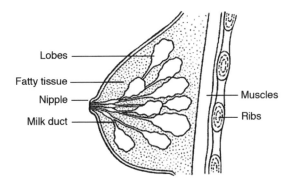

Lobes

Fatty tissue

Nipple

Milk duct

Muscles

Ribs

4. SOME OF THE RISK FACTORS

- Being a woman
- Getting older
- Getting your periods before 12 years old
- Having your menopause after age 50
- Never having children
- Having children after age 30
- Having had an abortion
- Family history
- Changes in the gene BRCA1/2 - Mutations inherited from parents
- Taking hormone replacement therapy (estrogen & progesterone)
- Taking birth control pills
- Prior personal history of breast cancer
- A prior biopsy from the breast showing atypical hyperplasia changes (LCIS)
- Not breastfeeding
- Drinking 2-5 alcoholic drinks per day
- Being Overweight
- Poor diet
- Living in a toxic environment
- Not exercising
- Stress

Self-examination

My gynecologist taught me how to do this at age 30, therefore I became familiar with my unique lumps and bumps which change during your menstrual cycle. Because of this, I was able to find my small tumor and went to see my doctor the next day. Remember, I had no pain.

In addition to new lumps or bumps in your breast, look for:

- Skin irritations or dimpling
- Nipple pain or nipples turning inward
- Redness or scaly areas on the nipple or breast skin
- A discharge from the nipple other than breast milk

Clinical breast examinations

My doctor performed this on the day I revealed my lump to her and this exam is part of your routine yearly exam. The doctor is trained to feel abnormalities and will then send you for further testing. Women after age 20 should have a clinical breast exam every year.

Mammogram

This is done by placing the breasts between plates for a few seconds while x-rays are taken. If something is found to be abnormal or your breast tissue is too dense, further testing is done. Sometimes tiny specks of calcium are detected and could be an early sign of cancer. Women over age 40 should get a mammogram yearly, however breast cancer is on the rise in younger women and I urge you to be proactive and get tested no matter what your age.

Diagnostic Mammogram

The breasts are placed on plates the same as a mammogram but the machinery is more advanced and able to afford better views and angles with magnification.

Ultrasound

This is a diagnostic test that uses sound waves to create images of tissues. Tissues of various densities reflect sound waves differently. You are positioned on a table with gel spread on your breast and a small wand is massaged over the gel. This is not a painful test, just a bit chilly from the gel. An ultrasound-assisted needle biopsy may also be ordered. This is when a needle is inserted into the lump with the ultra sound machine assisting the doctor and a small amount of tissue is removed and a biopsy is done.

Ductal Carcinoma in Situ (DCIS)
Also knows as intraductal carcinoma or non-invasive breast cancer, DCIS is confined to the ducts and has not yet spread. The numbers of new cases diagnosed in 2006 were around 65,000.

Invasive Ductal Cancer
Also called infiltrating ductal carcinoma, this type of breast cancer is the most common of all breast cancers and makes up about 70-80% of all new cases. It is found in the cells of the ducts and is usually a hard lump.

Mucinous Carcinoma (Colloid Carcinoma)
This accounts for 1-2% of all cases of invasive breast cancer formed by mucus-producing cancer cells. The prognosis for this type of breast cancer is usually better than for the other types.

Medullary Carcinoma
This type of breast cancer accounts for 5% of all breast cancers and involves a boundary between tumor tissue and normal tissue. It differs from other forms of invasive ductal breast cancers because it contains large cancer cells and immune system cells at the edges of the tumor. The prognosis for this type of breast cancer is usually better than for other invasive forms of breast cancer.

Tubular Carcinoma
This is characterized by tubular structures ringed with a single layer of cells. Only 2% of all breast cancers fall into this category.

Invasive Lobular Carcinoma
This form of breast cancer occurs at the ends of the ducts or in the lobules and accounts for about 25-30% of cases.

Paget's Disease

This form of breast cancer is rare and found in the ducts beneath the nipple and found in about 1% of all cases. This type of breast cancer usually starts with an itchy, eczema-like rash around the nipple. It is usually non-invasive.

Inflammatory Carcinoma

This aggressive type of breast cancer accounts for about 1-3% of all cases. The skin over the breasts appears to be inflamed or swollen because the skin's lymph vessels are blocked by cancer. It looks like an area of redness over the breasts.

If breast cancer is suspected, a biopsy is performed to obtain tissue to confirm the diagnosis. This is now more often done with a fine needle or core needle inserted through the skin into the tumor. If the tumor cannot be felt by your doctor and is only seen on the mammogram or ultrasound this same type of biopsy can be performed under the guidance of the mammogram (called a "stereotactic " biopsy) or the ultrasound. Sometimes a definite diagnosis cannot be made in this relatively non-invasive manner and an open surgery is performed by the doctor to remove part of or all of the tumor. Analysis is done to get a feeling of how aggressive the tumor is — to determine the "receptor status" and see if the tumor would respond to hormonal therapy. Hormonal therapy is more often used with postmenopausal women. Another important test checks if the cells in the tumor express a protein called Her2neu. These types of cancers are more aggressive but respond very well to a new medicine called Herceptin.

Additional tests such as chest x-rays, CT scans and blood work may be ordered depending on the size of the tumor. Staging is determined mainly by the size of the tumor and whether or not the cancer has spread to the lymph nodes or elsewhere in the body.

• **Stage 0**

Called carcinoma in situ, (DCIS) ductal carcinoma in situ or intraductal carcinoma (medical jargon for cancer). These cancers are early, limited to the cells in the lining of the lobules or ducts, have not invaded into the breast tissue and therefore cannot spread elsewhere. They are almost always curable with surgery. Note: LCIS (lobular carcinomas in-situ) is a misnomer. This is not cancer but is a risk factor for breast cancer in the future.

- Stage I

Early stage breast cancer where the tumor is less than 2 centimeters across and has not spread beyond the breast.

- Stage II

Early stage breast cancer where the tumor is either less than 2 centimeters and has spread to the lymph nodes under the arm; or the tumor is between 2 and 5 cm with or without spread to the lymph nodes under the arm or the tumor is greater than 5cm and has not spread outside the breast.

- Stage III

Locally advanced breast cancer where the tumor is greater than 5 centimeters across and has spread to the lymph nodes under the arm; or the cancer is extensive in the underarm lymph notes; or the cancer has spread to lymph nodes near the breastbone or the other tissues near the breast.

- Stage IV

Metastatic breast cancer where the cancer has spread outside the breast to other organs in the body.

Within these stages the tumor is also rated.

Option 1: Lumpectomy-BCT (breast conservation treatment), Segmental or Partial Mastectomy

All of these terms mean the same thing. Surgeons remove the tumor with a little bit of breast tissue around it or (if the tumor was removed previously) they remove a margin of tissue around the original site of the tumor. The surgeon may also dissect the lymph nodes under the arm so the pathologist can review them for signs of cancer. Most patients have a sentinel lymph node biopsy first to determine if a formal lymph node dissection is required. Most patients who have had lumpectomies are advised to follow their surgery with radiation therapy. Some patients opt not to have radiation or take drugs; instead they make dietary and lifestyle changes and follow a natural plan of care.

Option 2: Mastectomy

A removal of the entire breast. A Sentinel Node biopsy is also performed in this setting if the nodes are not already involved with the tumor. The patient may opt to have reconstruction done at the same time. (See chapter on reconstruction.) Despite the fact that the entire breast has been removed, there is always a risk of recurrence because there may be microscopic cancer cells that have spread to distant sites in the body. Most patients who have had a Mastectomy will not need radiation therapy, but some will. Note: Removing the entire breast does reduce the need for chemotherapy or hormone therapy.

Option 3: Radiation Therapy

Uses high-energy rays (similar to x-rays) to kill cancer cells. It comes from an external source and requires up to 6 weeks of treatments, 5 times per week. The treatment takes a few minutes and is painless. Newer techniques are being studied where the radiation therapy is delivered only to the part of the breast where the cancer is removed. This type of radiation is given over much shorter periods of time.

Option 4: Sentinel Node Biopsy

The sentinel node is found by injecting blue dye and/or a radioactive agent around the site of the tumor prior to surgery. The dye and radioactive material travel through the breast lymphatic vessels to the 1 or 2 lymph nodes that first drain from that part of the breast. A scan of the breast a few hours after being injected with the dye will show a picture of the route it took to get to the sentinel node. Using this technique, only a few nodes need to be removed to determine if cancer has spread. Removing many lymph nodes can be very painful in the short term and cause swelling of the arm in the long term (lymphedema). This test can hurt a bit. When the radioactive dye is being injected you will feel a stinging sensation.

Option 5: Chemotherapy

Uses anti-cancer drugs that go throughout the entire body. There are many different chemotherapy drugs and they are usually given in combinations approximately 3 to 6 months after you receive your surgery. Almost all of the chemotherapies have to be given through a vein. Other medications are given before or during to reduce some of the side effects of the chemotherapy. You will have to go to the doctor's office or clinic to receive the chemotherapy.

Option 6: Hormonal Therapy

An estrogen-blocking drug which taken in pill form for 5 years after your surgery. Two major categories of hormone therapy exist. The estrogen receptor blocking ones (Tamoxifen is most commonly used) and the drugs that block the production of estrogens made by the adrenal glands in post-menopausal women (aromitase inhibitors). This is prescribed when your tumor has been found to express estrogen and progesterone receptors. They can be taken during radiation therapy but should only be given after the entire chemotherapy course is completed if chemotherapy is needed. This is a personal decision and comes with side effects. Please discuss and understand all of your options.

Option 7: Biologic Therapy

If the pathologist finds the presence of HER-2/neu, which is a receptor that some breast cancers express, your chances are higher of having your cancer recur after surgery. Herceptin is a medication that blocks this receptor and when given with chemotherapy has proven to significantly reduce recurrence vs. chemotherapy alone. 30% of all breast cancers are HER-2 positive. Talk to your doctor and please do your homework on this one.

Follow-up Tests
After your surgery, it is recommended that you see your doctor every 3-4 months for the first year, then every 6 months for 4 years and once a year after 5 years have passed. During these visits, the doctor will examine you, run blood work and may order chest x-rays, mammograms or ultra-sound.

New techniques have made it possible for plastic surgeons to create a breast that looks natural and visually very close to what you were born with. Most reconstructions are carried out with the surgical oncologist performing the mastectomy with the goal of saving as much of the skin as possible, preserving the native skin envelope. Optimally, the plastic surgeon works in the same operative setting, performing the immediate reconstruction. This makes it possible for the patient to wake up from the surgery with a breast mound already in place, sparing them the trauma of seeing no breast at all while avoiding a second operation.

This is not a simple procedure and there are many options to discuss with your doctors to be sure the end result is in line with your expectations.

I would suggest that you meet with and interview the plastic surgeons that have worked with your doctor. The plastic surgeon will provide videos and written material which you should be sure to watch and read. In most cases they will have a list of references which includes women who you may speak with about their reconstruction experience. Remember, this is your body and you want to be sure to have all of the information possible to make the decision that is right for you. Almost all patients with early stage breast cancer are medically appropriate for reconstruction at the same time the breast is removed. The best candidates are those whose cancer can be eliminated by the mastectomy and will not need radiation after the mastectomy and are in good physical condition going into the surgery.

There are those that may opt to wait for a variety of reasons, some of which are:

- Because they need more time to weigh their options
- Because they do not want to have more than one surgery at the same time
- Doctors recommend they wait due to obesity, high blood pressure or smoking
- The breast may be reconstructed, performed in a more involved procedure using flaps of skin and other tissue.

Surgery does carry risks such as bleeding, fluid retention and scar tissue.

The ability of the plastic surgeon is not the only factor in achieving a good cosmetic outcome. The cancer surgeon plays a pivotal role in this endeavor by saving as much of the skin envelope as possible, as safety permits. This approach, referred to as a "skin sparing mastectomy", contributes greatly to the very important goal of preserving self image while at the same time treating the cancer.

Reconstruction Options:

Option 1: Skin Expansion
After the mastectomy is performed, the plastic surgeon inserts an implant to rebuild the breast. The surgeon will insert a balloon expander beneath your skin and chest muscle and then insert the implant. The implant shell is silicone filled with either silicone or a salt water called saline. Which option is best for you should be discussed with your oncologist and plastic surgeon. Some implants may require additional surgeries. Be sure to discuss these options with your doctor. Currently there is a clinical study using gel implants which you may be able to partake in. The FDA guidelines change regarding implants, therefore please do your homework.

Option 2: Flap Reconstruction

The surgeon will create a breast mound using your own skin and underlying attached soft tissue from areas such as the back, abdomen or buttock. This is called flap reconstruction. This type of surgery leaves scars where the tissue was removed and on the reconstructed breast and is a much more involved surgery.

Follow-up Procedures
Additional surgeries may be needed to enlarge, lift or reduce to create natural symmetrical breasts.

The nipple and the dark skin surrounding it, called the areola, are also reconstructed. This is done by using skin and tattoo techniques.

Self Examination

Although there is skepticism about the effectiveness of self-exams, it is what saved MY life! I found a tiny lump and went to see my gynecologist the next day. She agreed that it felt different than others I had found over the years and sent me for a mammogram which was negative. I then went to a surgeon for a needle biopsy, from which he was unable to draw any fluid so he suggested I wait until my next period. I insisted on a biopsy. Had I waited, the cancer would have had more time to grow inside of me.

Ultrasound

Most doctors will not recommend Ultrasound, but I believe it is the best test for young women and those with dense breast tissue. In most cases you will need to be proactive and ask for this test. Breast & Ovarian Cancer have been linked, therefore you may consider having an Ultrasound of the uterus as well for a base line. Ovarian cancer is a silent killer with virtually no symptoms. This test is worth the extra cost.

Blood Tests

As part of your regular blood work, please request:

• General Chemistry
• CA 125 Ovarian Carcinoma Associated Antigen
• CA 27.29 Breast Carcinoma Associated Antigen

Cutting Edge Tests
Mammastatin Serum Assay (MSA)

Based on an exclusive license from the University of Michigan; the assay measures the level of certain protein in blood serum. MSA technology has been studied for use as an aid in the risk assessment of breast cancer in women.

www.bio-diagnostics.com or 1-888-652-4246 for more information

Cadstream Advancing Breast MRI
Currently in use at over 50 centers nationwide, providing efficiency to expand imaging.
www.confirma.com

Breast Thermography
Medical Infrared Imaging has the ability to warn women up to 10 years before any other procedure that a cancer may be forming and it is non-invasive.
www.breastthermography.com

Did you know that 75% of women who get breast cancer have no family history?

Did you know that mammography is only 67% accurate?

Cancer prevention in general is really comprised of two approaches. The more common of the two is called "secondary prevention" – preventing deaths due to cancer by early diagnosis. Early detection programs specific to breast cancer have included a massive and effective public education effort, regularly scheduled appointments with primary care doctors or gynecologists, breast self-examination, and, of course, strict compliance to annual screening mammogram recommendations. Early detection has resulted in the single greatest impact on reducing deaths due to breast cancer.

"Primary prevention" efforts are aimed at actually reducing the incidence of a cancer within an identified risk group. Unfortunately, breast cancer is common in the general female population, a one in eight lifetime risk. Higher risk patients can be identified according to a variety of factors including age, menopausal status, age at first pregnancy, number of pregnancies, age of first menstrual period, use of birth control pills, high-fat content in diet, family history, a breast biopsy showing atypical hyperplasia or Lobular carcinoma in-situ (described earlier), and having one of the identified breast cancer genes (BRCA 1 or 2). Primary prevention efforts have included prophylactic mastectomies (removal of both breasts before cancer develops) and "chemoprevention" (taking medicines, particularly estrogen blocking agents).

Obviously, prophylactic mastectomies are way too radical to be used routinely and chemoprevention has side effects that otherwise healthy women with average risk should not be subjected to. However, in very high risk situations, one or the other may be considered. Mastectomies are only considered for the highest risk groups, women with a very strong family history and a biopsy showing atypical duct hyperplasia, or a biopsy showing LCIS or the presence of one of the breast cancer genes.

The availability of excellent breast reconstruction techniques has reduced some of the strong emotional response to such a radical approach. Prophylactic mastectomy is more effective than chemoprevention, but chemoprevention can reduce the risk for breast cancer by 50%. The current drug approved for breast cancer prevention is Tamoxifen for 5 years. A recent study, the results of which were only available in May of 2006, has shown that another estrogen blocking agent, Raloxifene (also known as Evista) is similar in its ability to prevent breast cancer and has less side effects.

- University of Texas, M.D. Anderson Cancer Center, Houston
  www.mdanderson.org

- Roswell Park Cancer Institute, Buffalo
  www.roswellpark.org

- Clarian Health Partners, Indianapolis
  www.clarian.org

- Memorial Sloan-Kettering Cancer Center, New York
  www.mskcc.org

- Johns Hopkins Hospital, Baltimore
  www.hopkinshospital.org

- Mayo Clinic, Rochester, Minnesota
  www.mayoclinic.org

- Duke University Medical Center, Durham, N.C.
  www.cancer.duke.edu

- University of Chicago Hospitals
  www.uchospitals.edu

- Massachusetts General Hospital, Boston
  www.mgh.harvard.edu

- UCLA Medical Center, Los Angeles
  www.healthcare.ucla.edu

FROM A TO Z TO HELP YOU AND ME

The words you will begin to hear ... and will need to understand.

A

ADENOMA
A benign tumor.

ADJUVANT
A substance that when added to a medicine speeds or improves its action.

ADJUVANT SYSTEMIC THERAPY
Treatment given in addition to surgery and radiation to eliminate microscopic tumors that may have spread to other sites. There are two types, chemotherapy and hormone therapy.

ALOPECIA
Hair loss.

ANESTHESIA
Loss of feeling or sensation. Local anesthesia may be introduced into a specific region of the body, such as the breast, by injection of a drug (a local anesthetic) into that area. General anesthesia involving the entire body may be induced through the vein.

ANEUPLOID (DNA Ploidy)
Presence of an abnormal number of chromosomes in cancer cells.

ANGIOGENESIS
Blood vessel formation, which usually accompanies the growth of malignant tissue.

ANTIBODY

A protein molecule produced by the immune system that specifically binds the antigen.

ANTICARCINOGEN

Referring to an agent that counteracts carcinogens (cancer causing agents).

ANTIEMETIC

A medicine to prevent or relieve nausea and vomiting.

ANTIGEN

Any of a variety of materials that induce the body's immune system to produce antibodies.

ANTIOXIDANT

Referring to an agent that counteracts oxidizing agents. Oxidizing agents are always present in the body and beneficial. However, when large amounts of oxidants are present in cells they can cause damage, especially to DNA that can lead to cancerous growth.

APOPTOSIS

A normal cellular process involving a genetically programmed series of events leading to the death of a cell.

AREOLA

The more darkly shaded circle of skin surrounding the nipple.

ASPIRATE

To remove fluid and a small number of cells.

ATYPICAL HYPERPLASIA

Overgrowth of mildly abnormal but non-cancerous (benign) cells within the breast milk ducts.

AXILLA

The underarm region.

AXILLARY DISSECTION
Surgical procedure to remove lymph nodes from under the arm.

AXILLARY LYMPH NODES
The lymph nodes under the arm.

AXILLARY SAMPLING (Axillary Dissection)
Removal of some or all of the lymph nodes in the armpit.

B

BACKGROUND
Usually refers to excess staining, beyond the intended target tissue.

B-CELLS
Type of white blood cells. Many B-cells mature into plasma cells which can produce antibody proteins necessary to fight off infections.

BENIGN
Not cancerous; does not invade nearby tissue or spread to other parts of the body.

BENIGN BREAST DISEASE
Non-cancerous conditions of the breast that can result in lumps or abnormalities on a mammogram. Examples include fluid-filled cysts and fibro adenoma.

BIOLOGICAL THERAPY
The use of the body's immune system, either directly or indirectly, to fight cancer or to lessen side effects that may be caused by some cancer treatments. Also known as immunotherapy, biotherapy or biological response modifier therapy.

BIOPSY
Removal of tissue which is then examined for cancer cells.

BONE SCAN
A test done to determine whether or not there are any signs of cancer in the bones. A small amount of radioactive material is injected into the bloodstream. It collects in the bones (especially abnormal areas) and is detected by a scanner.

BOOST
Additional dose of radiation to a reduced size radiation field.

BREAST CONSERVING SURGERY
Surgery that removes only part of the breast — the part containing and closely surrounding the cancer tumor.

BREAST SELF-EXAMINATION (BSE)
A method used by women to become familiar with the normal appearance and feel of their breast tissue so that if a change occurs it will be detected.

C

CACHEXIA
Loss of appetite and weight experienced by many cancer patients.

CALCIFICATIONS
Deposits of calcium in the breast that appear on a mammogram, and can sometimes indicate pre-cancerous or cancerous cell growth.

CANCER
General name for over 100 diseases in which cell growth is uncontrolled. A generic term for any kind of malignant tumor.

CENTIGRAY (Centigrays)
One centigray describes the amount of radiation absorbed by the

tissues and is equivalent to 100 RADs (doses of radiation).

CHEMOTHERAPY
A drug or combination of drugs given in cycles. These drugs kill cancer cells in various ways.

CLINICAL
Pertaining to the symptoms and course of a disease.

CLINICAL BREAST EXAMINATION (CBE)
The inspection and palpation of the breasts by a trained medical professional.

CLINICAL TRIALS
Research studies done with human patients. These studies generally test the benefits of possible new treatments or diagnostic procedures.

CORE NEEDLE BIOPSY
A needle biopsy using a wide-core needle with suction that removes pieces of tissue rather than just cells from a lump.

CYST
A closed cavity or sac that contains a liquid or semi-solid material.

CYTOLOGY
The study of cells.

CYTOPATHOLOGIST
A pathologist who specializes in looking at individual cells. A cytopathologist is needed to interpret the results of fine needle aspiration.

CYTOTOXICITY
Toxic or deadly. Killing cells or preventing their growth.

D

DEFINITIVE SURGERY
When all of the known tumor is removed and no follow-up surgery is needed.

DETOXIFICATION
The concept existing in many special regimens whereby the body is cleansed of unnatural and unhealthy agents.

DIAGNOSIS
The process for deciding what disease is present, using signs and symptoms.

DIAGNOSTIC MAMMOGRAM
A diagnostic mammogram is used to further evaluate a woman with a breast problem/symptom or an abnormal finding on a screening mammogram. This procedure involves two or more x-ray views per breast with higher magnification.

DIAGNOSTIC RADIOLOGIST
A physician who specializes in the diagnosis of diseases by the use of X-rays.

DIPLOID (DNA Ploidy)
Having two sets of chromosomes; one set from each parent.

DISTANT RECURRENCE
Return of cancer that has spread to other parts of the body, such as the lungs, liver, or bone.

DNA
Deoxyribonucleic acid. The biochemical make-up of chromosomes.

DOXORUBICIN
An antibiotic used as an anti-cancer drug.

DUCT
A pathway in the breast through which milk passes from lobes to the nipple.

DUCTAL CARCINOMA IN SITU (DCIS)
Type of in situ (non-invasive) breast cancer that originates mainly in the milk ducts of the breast.

DUCTAL PAPILLOMA
A non-cancerous breast tumor, arising in the breast duct that usually cannot be felt. It generally appears as either a bloody or clear nipple discharge.

E

ENDOCRINE MANIPULATION (Hormone Therapy)
Treating the breast cancer by changing the hormonal balance of the body instead of using cell-killing drugs.

ESTROGEN (also oestrogen)
A female hormone produced by the ovaries and adrenal glands, important to reproduction, and which may stimulate some cancers

ESTROGEN RECEPTORS
A protein which specifically binds to estrogen and mediates its biological activity. When present in breast cancer, it predicts response to hormonal therapy.

EXCISIONAL BIOPSY
Surgical procedure that removes the entire suspicious area (plus some surrounding normal tissue) from the breast. Also called lumpectomy, partial mastectomy, or segmental mastectomy.

EXTERNAL BEAM RADIATION (Radiation Therapy)
A process of delivering high-energy radiation via a treatment machine (linear accelerator) using electron or photon beams.

F

FALSE NEGATIVE
A test result that incorrectly reports that a person is disease-free when they actually have the disease.

FALSE POSITIVE
Test result that incorrectly reports a healthy person has a disease.

FAT NECROSIS
A non-cancerous breast change in which the breast responds to trauma with a firm, irregular mass, often years after the event. The mass is the result of fatty tissue dying, following either surgery, or blunt trauma to the breast. This breast change is not associated with an increased risk to breast cancer.

FIBROADENOMA
A benign fibrous tumor that may occur at any age but is more common in young adulthood.

FIBROCYSTIC CONDITION (Fibrocystic changes)
Non-cancerous breast condition, sometimes resulting in painful cycle cysts or lumpy breasts, also referred to as benign breast disease.

FINE NEEDLE ASPIRATION (FNA)
Specimen acquired through insertion of a thin needle used to remove a sample of cells from the abnormal area of the breast. Also called fine needle.

FLOW CYTOMETRY
A laboratory test performed on malignant breast tissue to determine the growth rate of malignant cells and the presence of abnormal chromosomes.

FROZEN SECTION
Immediate freezing of biopsied tissue for analysis by the pathologist to find out if it is malignant (cancerous) or benign (not cancerous).

G

GALACTOCELE
A clogged milk duct.

GENE
The part of a person's cells that contains all the DNA information that determines how they will grow and develop, and how their body works. The information in a person's genes is inherited from previous generations on both sides of a person's family.

GENE MUTATION
A mistake or alteration of the information contained in a gene.

GENERAL PRACTITIONER/INTERNIST
A woman's personal or family physician that may first detect a suspicious area through clinical breast exam or abnormal mammogram.

GERSON DIET
Developed in the 1940s by German physician Max Gerson, focusing on restoring metabolic balance to the body through organic, vegetarian diet, enemas and calf's liver.

H

HER2/NEU (also called erbB2)
Oncoprotein (product of an oncogene); over expression is a negative prognostic indicator in many cancers, including breast and ovarian carcinoma. It may also be a good predictor of which women may respond to certain chemotherapy and antibody treatments.

HISTOGRAM
Two-dimensional graph of data (i.e., content vs. cell number).

HOMEOPATHY
The art of curing founded on resemblances. Theory and practice is that the disease is cured by remedies which produce effects similar to the symptoms. Founded in Europe by Dr. Samuel Hahnemann in the 1800's.

HORMONE
Chemicals produced by various glands in the body, which produce specific effects on specific target organs and tissues.

HORMONE RECEPTORS
Specific proteins in breast cells that hormones attach to. A high number of hormone receptors often indicate that a cancer cell needs the hormone to grow.

HORMONE THERAPY
Treatment that works by keeping cancer cells from getting the hormones they need to grow.

I

IMAGE ANALYZER
Instrument consisting of a microscope, camera and computer used to quantify cellular components that have been marked or stained.

IMMUNOHISTOCHEMISTRY (IHC)
Technique that uses antibodies to identify and mark antigens expressed by cells in tissue.

IMMUNOTHERAPY
Treatment that uses the body's natural defenses to fight cancer. Also called biological therapy.

IMPLANT (Breast)
An "envelope" containing silicone, saline or both, used to restore breast form.

INCIDENCE
The number of new cases of a disease that develop in a specific time period.

INCISIONAL BIOPSY
Surgical biopsy that removes only part of the tumor, usually done on advanced or large tumors.

INDUCTION CHEMOTHERAPY
(also know as Primary Chemotherapy, Preoperative Chemotherapy, or Neoadjuvant Therapy)
Chemotherapy used as a first treatment, often used for large or advanced cancers to shrink tumors before surgery.

INFORMED CONSENT (Risks and Benefits)
The process through which a patient learns about the possible benefits and side effects of a recommended treatment plan and then accepts or declines the treatment. The patient is usually asked to sign a consent document, and may decide to stop the treatment at any time and can receive other available medical care.

IN SITU
In the natural or normal place, confined to the site or origin without invasion of neighboring tissues.

IN SITU CANCER
Cancers contained in the milk ducts and lobules of the breast that have not left their original location and spread to the surrounding breast tissue. In situ means "in place."

INTRADUCTAL
Within the milk duct. Intraductal can describe a benign or malignant process.

INTRADUCTAL HYPERPLASIA
An excess of cells growing within the breast's milk ducts.

INTRAVENOUS
Being within or entering the body by way of the veins.

INVASIVE CANCER
Cancer that has spread from the original location into the surrounding breast tissue and possibly into the lymph nodes and other parts of the body.

INVESTIGATIONAL NEW DRUG
(New Experimental Treatment)
A chemical or biological drug that has been approved for use by clinical investigators in research trials but which is not yet available for commercial use.

L

LACTATION
The process of producing milk and breastfeeding a child.

LACTIC ACID
Syrupy, water soluble liquid produced as waste by cancer cell metabolism.

LARGE VEINS OR DEEP VEINS
The large veins deep inside the legs that carry blood from the lower limbs back to the heart.

LESIONS
Area of abnormal tissue.

LINEAR ACCELERATOR
The device used during radiation therapy to direct X-rays into the body.

LOBULAR CARCINOMA IN SITU (LCIS)
An in situ cancer where the cells originate mainly in the lobules of the breast.

LOBULES
Spherical-shaped sacs in the breast that produce milk.

LOCAL ANESTHETIC
Anesthesia that only numbs the cells in a specific area.

LOCAL TREATMENT
Treatment that focuses on getting rid of the cancer from a limited (local) area, namely the breast, the chest wall, and lymph nodes under the arm pit (axillary nodes).

LOCALIZED BREAST CANCER
Cancer that is contained in the breast and has not spread to surrounding tissue, lymph nodes, or other organs.

LUMP
Any kind of mass in the breast or elsewhere in the body.

LUMPECTOMY
The surgical removal of only the cancerous breast lump. This type of surgery is usually followed by radiation therapy.

LYMPHATIC SYSTEM
The network of lymph glands and vessels throughout the body.

LYMPHEDEMA
Fluid accumulation that causes swelling which may arise from surgery to remove lymph nodes or radiation.

LYMPH NODES OR LYMPH GLANDS
Small clumps of immune cells scattered along the path of the lymphatic system. They produce and store white blood cells and filter harmful substances out. They are found in the underarms, groin, neck, chest and abdomen.

M

MACROBIOTICS
Dietary therapy based on the concepts of yin and yang; encourages largely vegetarian, organic foods and defines specific methods of preparation.

MALIGNANT
Cancerous.

MAMMARY DUCT
Ducts or canals (about 15-20), that carry milk from the lobules to the nipple opening when a woman is breastfeeding.

MAMMARY DUCT ECTASIA
A non-cancerous breast condition resulting from the inflammation and enlargement of the ducts behind the nipple. Generally women do not experience any symptoms; however, calcifications seen on a mammogram may indicate its presence. No treatment is necessary if the woman is not experiencing any symptoms (burning, pain or itching of the nipple area).

MAMMARY GLANDS (Breast Tissue)
The breast glands that produce and carry milk, by way of ducts, to the nipples during pregnancy.

MAMMOGRAM
An x-ray of the breast.

MARGINS
The area of normal tissue surrounding the cancerous tumor after it has been removed during surgery. A margin is uninvolved (also known as clean or negative) if there is only normal tissue (and no cancer cells) at the edges of the tissue removed. Uninvolved margins indicate that the entire tumor was removed. With involved (also known as dirty or positive) margins, normal tissue does not completely surround the tumor, and therefore the entire tumor was not removed.

MASTECTOMY
Surgical removal of the breast and some surrounding tissue.

MASTITIS
An inflammation of the breast. Symptoms include pain, nipple discharge, fever and redness and/or hardness over an area of the breast.

MELATONIN
Hormone produced by the pineal gland in the brain and an important part of the body's internal timing system.

MENARCHE
The first menstrual period.

MENOPAUSE
The ending of the normal menstrual cycle in women. It occurs most frequently in the late forties or early fifties.

METABOLIZED
The chemical process whereby drugs and food are broken down by the body.

METASTASES
Spread of cancer to other organs through the lymphatic and/or circulatory system.

MICROCALCIFICATIONS
Small clustered deposits of calcium in the breast, which may be seen on a mammogram. These may or may not be associated with a breast lump. Approximately 20-25% represent breast cancer.

MICROMETASTASES
Presence of a small number of tumor cells, particularly in the lymph nodes and bone marrow, not readily detected by standard methods.

MODIFIED RADICAL MASTECTOMY (Total Mastectomy)
Most common type of mastectomy performed today. The breast skin, nipple, areola and underarm lymph nodes are removed, while the chest muscles are saved.

MONOCLONAL ANTIBODY
Immune proteins that can locate and bind to cancer cells wherever they are in the body. They can be used alone, or they can be used to deliver drugs, toxins, or radioactive material directly to tumor cells.

MRI (Magnetic Resonance Imaging)
An imaging technique that uses a magnet linked to a computer to create detailed pictures of parts of the body like the liver, brain, lung, chest, or any other organs suspected of having metastases.

MULTIFOCAL TUMORS
Multiple tumors.

MULTIMODALITY THERAPY (Combination of Surgery)
Use of two or more treatment methods (i.e., surgery, radiation therapy, chemotherapy, immunotherapy) in combination or sequentially to achieve optimal results.

N

NEEDLE-LOCALIZATION (also known as Wire Localization)
Insertion of a very thin wire into an abnormal area of the breast, used to highlight the location of a nonpalpable lesion so that is can be removed during open biopsy or breast conserving surgery.

NEOADJUVANT THERAPY
Chemotherapy or hormone therapy used as a first treatment, often to shrink large or advanced cancers before surgery.

NEOPLASIA
Abnormal or new growth.

NEOPLASM
Excessive number of cells in a mass that can be either benign or malignant.

NONPALPABLE
Breast lumps or abnormalities that cannot be felt but may be detected by a mammogram, sonogram or MRI.

O

ONCOGENE
Abnormal genes that convert a cell into a tumor cell and associated with many cancers.

ONCOLOGIST
The doctor responsible for planning and overseeing drug treatment of cancer, such as chemotherapy and hormone therapy.

- Medical Oncologist—A physician specializing in the treatment of cancer using Chemotherapy.
- Radiation Oncologist—A physician specializing in the treatment of cancer using high-energy X-rays.
- Surgical Oncologist—A physician specializing in the treatment of cancer using surgical procedures.

ONCOLOGY
The study of diseases that cause cancer.

ONE-STEP PROCEDURE (Frozen Sections)
A method for diagnosis and treatment of breast cancer. The biopsy is performed under general anesthesia. If cancer is confirmed by frozen section examination, a surgeon will then proceed with definitive surgical treatment. It should be noted that this is no

longer the standard procedure unless the woman is informed and consents in advance to a one-step procedure.

OOPHORECTOMY
Surgical removal of the ovaries.

ORGANELLE
A structurally discrete component of a cell.

P

P53
A tumor suppresser gene. Mutations in the P53 gene are associated with many different cancers, and are related to cancer progression.

PALLIATIVE THERAPY (Palliation)
A treatment that may relieve symptoms without curing the disease such as chemotherapy, radiation or surgery.

PALPABLE MASS
Breast lumps or abnormalities that can be felt during a clinical breast exam.

PALPATION
A simple technique in which a doctor presses lightly on the surface of the body to feel the organs and tissues underneath.

PARTIAL MASTECTOMY
(Breast Conserving Therapy, Lumpectomy, Wide Excision or Excisional Biopsy)
Surgery that removes only the part of the breast containing and closely surrounding the cancer tumor.

PATHOLOGIST
The doctor who microscopically evaluates the breast tissue and lymph nodes removed during biopsy or surgery.

PATHOLOGY
The branch of medicine which studies structural and functional changes in tissues and organs of the body which cause or are caused by disease.

PERMANENT SECTION (Standard Analysis)
A method used for final tissue diagnosis. After overnight tissue processing, thin slices of tissue are mounted on a slide and examined microscopically by a pathologist. These sections are of better quality than the frozen section, and are used for final pathological diagnosis. It generally takes three working days to receive this final pathology report.

PITUITARY GLAND
The part of the brain that regulates growth and other glands in the body, such as the ovaries.

PREDICTIVE FACTORS
Factors, such as hormone receptor status, that help predict the kind of treatment that will be most effective for a specific cancer case.

PREDISPOSE
To make more susceptible to a disease.

PREMENOPAUSAL WOMEN
Women who are having regular periods.

PREOPERATIVE CHEMOTHERAPY
Chemotherapy used as first treatment, often used for large or advanced tumors.

PRIMARY TUMOR
The original cancer in the breast.

PROGESTERONE RECEPTOR
Specific protein that binds to progesterone and mediates its biological activity.

PROGNOSIS

The expected or probable outcome or course of a disease; the chance of recovery.

PROGNOSTIC FACTORS

Factors, such as tumor type, size, and grade that help to determine a woman's prognosis.

PROLIFERATION

Cell cycle kinetics, reproduction or multiplication of a cell.

PROPHYLACTIC (PREVENTIVE) MASTECTOMY

A procedure sometimes recommended for a patient at high risk of developing cancer in one or both breasts. Breast tissue is removed without removing skin or muscle.

PROSTHESIS (Breast)

An artificial breast form that can be worn under clothing after a mastectomy.

PROTOCOL

An outline or plan for use of an experimental drug, treatment or procedure in cancer therapy or diagnosis.

Q

QUADRANTECTOMY

In this surgical procedure, one quadrant or ¼ of the breast is removed. A separate incision is made for the axillary dissection.

R

RAD (Dose of Radiation)

Abbreviation for "radiation absorbed dose." This term describes the amount of radiation absorbed by the tissues and is equal to one centigray.

RADIATION ONCOLOGIST
The doctor responsible for planning and overseeing radiation therapy.

RADIATION THERAPY (Radiotherapy)
Treatment given by a radiation oncologist using moderate-dose radiation to kill or damage cancer cells in the area exposed.

RADICAL MASTECTOMY (Halsted Radical)
The surgical removal of the breast, chest muscles, and underarm lymph nodes.

RADIOLOGIST
Specialist who oversees and reads any X-rays, mammograms, or other scans related to diagnosis or follow-up.

RECONSTRUCTION
A way to recreate the shape of a breast after the natural breast has been removed. Various procedures are available, some of which involve the use of implants. May also be referred to as reconstruction mammoplasty.

RECURRENCE
Return of cancer in the same site or another location.

REGRESSION
The shrinking of a tumor.

REMISSION
A temporary or permanent disappearance of the signs and symptoms of cancer.

RISK
Probability of disease developing in an individual during a specified time period.

RISK-BENEFIT RATIO (Risks and Benefits)
The relationship between the possible (or expected) side effects and benefits of a recommended treatment or procedure.

RNA
A nucleic acid found in living cells that plays a role in transferring information from DNA to the protein-forming system of a cell.

S

SARCOMA
A malignant cancer that arises in the supportive tissues such as bone, cartilage, fat or muscle.

SCREENING
A test or procedure used to detect cancer or pre-cancerous condition in an apparently healthy person without symptoms.

SCREENING MAMMOGRAM
Used to identify early signs of breast cancer in a woman who is not currently having any breast problems or symptoms. This procedure involves two x-ray views of the breast.

SECOND PRIMARY TUMOR
In a woman who has had breast cancer, it is a second breast cancer that may arise in a different location from the first. In a local recurrence, the tumor recurs near the location of the primary tumor.

SENSITIVITY
In IHC (Immuno Histo Chemistry), the ability of an antibody to detect the presence of an antigen, particularly at low antigen levels.

SENTINEL NODE BIOPSY
The surgical removal and examination of a single axillary node (the sentinel node or first node filtering lymph fluid from the tumor site) to see if the node contains cancer cells.

SERUM
Fluid component of blood (noncellular).

SIMULATOR (for Radiation Therapy)
A clinical X-ray unit used to define the exact treatment area for radiation therapy.

SONOGRAM
Diagnostic test that uses sound waves to create images of tissues and organs. Tissues of different densities reflect sound waves differently.

SPECIMEN
Material sent in for evaluation, biopsy (tissue) or cell suspensions (body fluids).

S-PHASE FRACTION
Examination of cancer cells to see how many are in the process of dividing DNA at any one time.

STAGING
Certain tests and examinations done before any type of definitive treatment to determine if the cancer has spread.

STAINING
Use of a dye or reagents (substance used to detect or measure another substance) to produce color in the tissue or microorganisms for microscopic examination.

STANDARD TREATMENT
The usual treatment currently in widespread use and considered to be of proven effectiveness on the basis of previous experience.

STEREOTACTIC BREAST BIOPSY
(Stereo Tactic Mammography)
A core needle biopsy performed with use of stereo tactic mammography.

STEREOTACTIC MAMMOGRAPHY
Three-dimensional mammography used when taking a needle biopsy of a nonpalpable lesion.

SURGICAL ONCOLOGIST
A physician specializing in the treatment of cancer using surgical procedures.

SYSTEMIC TREATMENT
Treatment of the whole body with substances that travel through the bloodstream and affect cancer cells all over the body.

T

TAMOXIFEN
A drug that is used to treat both early and advanced stage breast cancer. It works by blocking the hormone estrogen from cancer cells that are estrogen receptor-positive, therefore preventing their growth. Taken in pill form.

TAXOL
A chemotherapeutic agent derived from the bark of the yew tree, with anti-tumor agents.

THERAPEUTIC TOUCH
Process whereby trained practitioners enter a semi-meditative state and hold their hands just above the body to sense energy imbalances due to illness. Healing energy is then transferred to the patient.

TUMOR
An abnormal growth or mass of tissue which may be benign (non-cancerous) or malignant (cancerous).

TUMOR GRADE (Low, Medium, or High)
Describes how closely a cancer resembles normal tissue. The higher the grade, the less it resembles normal tissue, and the faster the cancer's rate of growth is likely to be.

TUMOR SUPPRESSER GENE
A gene involved in the normal growth regulation of cells. Abnormalities (mutations) of tumor suppresser genes are associated with the cause and progression of cancer based on abnormal cell growth.

TWO-STEP PROCEDURE
Surgical biopsy and breast surgery performed in two separate surgeries.

U

ULTRASOUND
Diagnostic test that uses sound waves to create images of tissues and organs. Tissues of different densities reflect sound waves differently.

W

WEDGE EXCISION (BREAST CONSERVING SURGERY)
This surgical procedure involves the removal of a portion of the breast tissue — the amount not specified. It is important that the woman clarify with her surgeon the extent of breast tissue to be removed.

WIRE-LOCALIZATION
Insertion of a very thin wire into an abnormal area of the breast, used to highlight the location of a nonpalpable lesion so that is can be removed during open biopsy or breast conserving surgery.

X

X-RAYS
Radiation that can be useful, at low levels, in the diagnosis of cancer and, at high levels, in its treatment.

www.cancerdecisions.com

If you have just been diagnosed with cancer, this is an incredible resource. Dr. Ralph Moss, a leading consultant on cancer, addresses each request with commitment and offers expert advice for patients and their families on the best alternative, complementary and conventional options for specific types of cancer. Call 800-980-1234 to order your personal Moss Report.

www.drday.com

Dr. Lorraine Day reversed her severe advanced cancer by rebuilding her immune system through natural therapies, allowing her body to heal itself. She is an internationally acclaimed orthopedics trauma surgeon and best-selling author who was on the faculty at University of California, San Francisco, School of Medicine as Associate Professor and Vice Chairman of Department of Orthopedics for 15 years. Dr. Day has lectured extensively in the US and has been on 60 Minutes, Nightline, CNN Crossfire, Oprah Winfrey, and Larry King.

www.healthywomen.org

The not-for-profit National Women's Health Resource Center (NWHRC) is the leading independent information source for women. NWHRC develops and distributes up-to-date and objective women's health information based on the latest advances in medical research practice. The NWHRC believes that all women should have access to trusted and reliable health information.

www.thecancer.net

The Cancer Information Network is loaded with information and cutting edge cancer news.

www.komen.org

The Susan G. Komen Breast Cancer Foundation was founded in 1978 as a result of a promise between two sisters. Susan died at age 36 years and her sister Nancy made a promise to do everything possible to eradicate breast cancer through research, education, screening and treatment. For 20 years this foundation has been a global leader in the fight against breast cancer. Innovative research and community-based outreach programs were made possible by a network of US and International Affiliates and events like The Race for the Cure. You can search on this site and sign up for a free e-newsletter.

www.thebreastsite.com

Your guide to breast health, products, services and information developed with one purpose – to give users up-to-date information on a variety of areas related to breast health. This site offers a very good book store and other related links.

www.nationalbreastcancer.org

Help for today...hope for tomorrow. The founder of this site is Janelle Hail, a survivor of 25 years, who relates to women with compassion, understanding and inspiration. She speaks across the nation at associations, organizations, women's groups and homeless shelters with the goal of educating women about breast cancer.

www.cancer.com

This is a comprehensive web site listing credible websites for all those whose lives are touched by cancer.

www.mdanderson.org

The virtual home of The Nellie B. Connally Breast Clinic—one of the best in the world. This is where I went for my surgery. This website affords up-to-date information on breast cancer options and support groups. The University of Texas M. D. Anderson Cancer Center is a very welcoming, warm and efficient hospital.

www.medical-dictionary.com

Definitions of words related to the medical field.

www.cancer.org

The American Cancer Society is a nationwide community-based voluntary health organization headquartered in Atlanta, Georgia. The ACS has state divisions and more than 3,400 local offices and over 2 million volunteers. Dedicated to eliminating cancer as a major health problem by saving lives and diminishing suffering, it is active in research, education, advocacy and service.

www.drmcdougall.com

John McDougall, founder of The McDougall Plan for Healthy Living, has been studying and writing on the effects of nutrition on diseases for over 30 years. Dr. McDougall believes that we should all look and feel good and enjoy optimal health for a lifetime.

www.homeopathic.org

The National Center for Homeopathy website offers a wealth of information. This medical system originated in Europe two hundred years ago and can effectively treat many diseases including breast cancer. The site also offers a global practitioners guide.

www.nccam.nih.gov

The National Center for Complementary and Alternative Medicine at the National Institute of Health. This site lists things to know about evaluating diseases and an A to Z guide on disease treatments and conditions.

www. breastcanceralliance.org

Founded in 1996 by Mary Waterman who was diagnosed with stage four breast cancer. Mary knew her chances for long-term survival were not good and wanted to help other women fight breast cancer through research, health, education, and most importantly, early detection. Mary died in 1996 but her mission and vision continue to inspire many. The Breast Cancer Alliance has raised over 7 million dollars since 1996 to fund innovative breast cancer research and to promote breast health. They are the 7th largest non-profit, private funding provider of breast cancer research in the U.S. Near and dear to me, they are headquartered in my hometown of Greenwich, CT.

www.weSpark.org

weSpark is a special site to visit, founded by Wendie Jo Sperber, an actress, mother and breast cancer survivor. Wendie's dream was to help those affected by cancer by providing a home-like setting where they could share their experience, strength and hope free of charge. In the fall of 2001, weSpark opened in Sherman Oaks, California. This website is a testimony to Wendie's determination and hard work. Wendie recently passed away but I had the opportunity to speak with her and I was very moved by her words and her heart.

www.bcrfcure.org

The Breast Cancer Research Foundation was founded by Evelyn Lauder who raised 18 million dollars in a fund drive between 1989 and 1992. The site for the Evelyn H. Lauder Breast Center at Memorial Sloan-Kettering, which offers survivor profiles, Breast Health Library, research information, support and events. The mission of this not-for-profit organization is to achieve prevention and cures by providing critical funding for innovative clinical and genetic research at leading medical centers, while increasing awareness.

www.EIFoundation.org

Entertainment Industry Foundation responds to some of the most critical needs facing our society. EIF helps raise awareness and funds to causes such as childhood hunger, cancer research, and much more. A special fundraising event of EIF is the Revlon Run/ Walk for Women.

www.revlonrunwalk.com

Created in 1993 by cancer activist Lily Tartikoff, Revlon Chairman Ronald O. Perelman and the Entertainment Industry Foundation, the Revlon Run/Walk has grown into the nations largest 5K event for women challenged with breast and ovarian cancer. Since 1993, 25 million has been raised.

www.gildasclub.org

Gilda's Club is a cancer support community where men, women and children, who have any type of cancer, at any stage can come together with friends for free social and emotional support.

www.ivanhoe.com

Ivanhoe Broadcast News, the country's largest television organization covers medical breakthroughs. Located in Orlando, FL and founded by Marjorie Bekaert Thomas & Bette BonFleur.

Many cancers can result in part from some malfunction of the immune system. This includes, breast, prostrate, leukemia, melanoma, lymphoma, brain cancer, cancers of the blood, stomach, colon and more.

Your immune system and your liver are working together to fight off disease from the time you were born. The cells of your immune system work in the tens of millions against any site of infection to kill it off. These cells have guards posted to spot the first signs of trouble with a communication network that decides how to proceed and when to multiply. This highly aggressive group of cells can destroy malignant cells.

Your immune system is equipped to fight all threats, but you must feed it with nutrients and antioxidants. The average cell suffers 10,000 free-radical assaults per day.

Your immune system is your friend, and your own private army and ally against disease and danger. It has been demonstrated repeatedly in both animals and human studies that dietary changes can actually reverse pre-malignant changes in many sites in the body. Cells that have begun to turn cancerous can return to normal function if the body is taking in nutrients through diet.

Cancer is serious business, but don't be pressured to make decisions. Take your time to evaluate the best treatment options for you. In the best possible world your oncologist and primary care physician will be cordial colleagues; teamed with skilled herbalists, nutritionists, support group leaders and spiritual organizations. A team that complements one another will understand your emotional and physical needs.

Explore your options!

Over 80% of most cancers have environmental origins.

Your personal choices, lifestyle and eating habits fit in the category of environmental factors.

The remaining factors include pollutants in our air, toxic chemicals in our food and water, cosmetic pesticides, electromagnetic field exposure in our homes and workplaces and other synthetic substances that are foreign to nature and should be avoided.

Research environmental issues in your own community. You might be surprised to find potential risks on your own street or in your home.

A recent article I read states that according to tests conducted on 230 soft drinks in Britain and France, high levels of benzene, a compound known to cause cancer have been detected. Traces of this carcinogenic chemical found in soft drinks is at eight times the level permitted in drinking water. This was reported by www.timesonline.co.uk, March 2, 2006.

What's in your drinking water and soft drinks?

Get involved in your own community.

Be informed.

Help yourself, your family and your friends.

Antiperspirants contain chemicals and toxins that are absorbed into your body in your armpit area and may cause a concentration of toxins that lead to cell mutations.

Think about it logically. We shave this area frequently, and apply antiperspirants daily. Please check the ingredients in the product you are currently using and you decide.

Please steer clear of any products that list aluminum.

There are many natural and effective products on the market.

The human body has a few areas that it uses to purge toxins: behind the knees, behind the ears, the groin area, and the armpits. The toxins are purged in the form of perspiration. Antiperspirant, as the name clearly indicates, prevents you from perspiring, thereby inhibiting the body from purging toxins. These toxins do not just magically disappear. Instead the body deposits them. With the armpits blocked, this could happen in the lymph nodes, closest to the armpit.

A high percentage of breast cancer tumors are found in the upper outside quadrant of the breast area because about 80% of breast tissue is located in that area. This is also where the lymph nodes are located. Additionally, men are less likely (but not completely exempt), to develop breast cancer prompted by antiperspirant usage because most of the product is caught in the hair located in their armpits and not directly applied to the skin.

Women who apply antiperspirant right after shaving increase the risk further because shaving may cause nicks in the skin, which aid in the chemicals entering into the body from the armpit area.

The bottom line: Sweating is good…cancer is not!

It is as important to use non-toxic body care products as it is to eat healthy, pesticide-free foods. You will be surprised to find that even products that claim to be healthy or natural may include some of these harmful ingredients.

Aubrey Organics is a great source for toxic-free products for your body, hair, skin and home. Their newest product, launched in September 2002, is organic hair color for brunettes. They are working to expand this line to include all hair colors.

Aubrey Hampton, CEO of Aubrey Organics has generoulsy offered use of this list.
Visit www.AubreyOrganics.com to order these amazing products that smell great!

Imidazolidinyl Urea and Diazolidinyl Urea

These are the most commonly used preservatives after the parabens. They are well established as a primary cause of contact dermatitis. Two trade names for these chemicals are Germall II and Germall 115. Germall 115 releases formaldehyde at just over 10 degrees.

Methyl and Propyl and Butyl and Ethyl Paraben

Used as inhibitors of microbial growth and to extend shelf life of products. Widely used even though they are known to be toxic. They have caused allergic reactions and skin rashes.

Petrolatum
You will find this in many lip products claiming to aid in sunburn and chapping. Petrolatum is a mineral oil jelly, and causes a lot of problems when used on the skin. It increases photosensitivity (i.e., promotes sun damage), and tends to interfere with the body's own natural moisturizing mechanism, leading to dry skin and chapping. Using products with petrolatum will create the very conditions it claims to alleviate. Manufacturers use petrolatum because it is unbelievably cheap.

Propylene Glycol
Ideally, this is a vegetable glycerin mixed with grain alcohol, both of which are natural. Usually it is a synthetic petrochemical mix used as a humectant which has been known to cause allergic reactions.

PVP/VA Copolymer
A petroleum-derived chemical used in hair sprays, wave sets and other cosmetics.

Sodium Lauryl Sulfate
This synthetic substance is used in shampoos for its detergent and foam-building abilities. It causes eye irritations, skin rashes, hair loss, scalp scurf similar to dandruff and allergic reactions. It is frequently disguised in pseudo-natural cosmetics with the parenthetic explanation, "comes from coconut."

Stearalkonium Chloride
A chemical used in hair conditioners and creams that causes allergic reactions. Stearalkonium chloride was developed by the fabric industry as a fabric softener, and is a lot cheaper and easier to use in hair conditioning formulas than proteins or herbals, which do help hair health.

Synthetic Colors
The synthetic colors used to make a cosmetic "pretty" should be avoided at all costs. They will be labeled as FD&C or D&C, followed by a color and a number. Example: FD&C Red No.6 / D&C Green No. 6.

Synthetic Fragrances
The synthetic fragrances used in cosmetics can have as many as 200 ingredients. There is no way to know what the chemicals are, since on the label it will simply say "Fragrance". Some of the problems caused by these chemicals are headaches, dizziness, rash, hyper-pigmentation, coughing, and skin irritation.

Triethanolamine
Often used in cosmetics to adjust the pH level, and used with many fatty acids to convert acid to salt (stearate), which then becomes the base, for a cleanser. TEA causes allergic reactions including eye problems, dryness of hair and skin and could be toxic if absorbed into the body over a long period of time.

Please look at the ingredients in the products you purchase.

Vitamin A/Beta-Carotene

An antioxidant that prevents free radical damage and is thought to help the body fight cancer and heart disease. Vitamin A supports eye and skin health, bone growth, and supports immunity.

Vitamin C (Ascorbic Acid)

An antioxidant which may reduce the risk of cancer, protects organs, enhances the immune system, lowers LDL (bad) cholesterol, fights skin damage, protects DNA, and helps make collagen.

Vitamin D

Increases calcium absorption which supports strong bones, and is an immune system regulator. We need more Vitamin D as we age. Vitamin D is produced in the skin with the presence of sunshine.

Vitamin E – 100% Natural Mixed Tocopherols
A major antioxidant particularly important in protecting the body's cells from free radical damage, inhibits cancer, lowers heart disease risk, protects DNA, improves blood flow to extremities, and helps raise HDL (good) cholesterol.

B VITAMINS

B1 (thiamin)

Supports the appetite, nerves, function of heart muscle cells, allows the body to properly use carbohydrates and protein, and improves mental sharpness.

B2 (riboflavin)

Essential for energy generation, supports skin & eye health, and heart muscle function.

B3 (niacin)

Assists in chemical reactions within the body, supports healthy functioning of the nervous and digestive systems, lowers LDL (bad) cholesterol and helps fight fatigue.

B6 (pyridoxine)

Makes red blood cells, assists in protein and fat metabolism.

B12 (cobalamin)

Helps make new cells and protects nerves. We need more B12 as we age.

Do you take a multivitamin every day? If the answer is yes, you might be surprised to learn that what your are taking is not enough. Please take the time to research the best for you and your body. My favorite is Eco-Green by Now.

Water is your friend!

The first thing I do every morning is drink a large 24 oz. bottle of water. Every function of the body is monitored by the efficient flow of water. Every system in your body, from brain to bowel, depends on water.

Water regulates your body temperature, transports nutrients and oxygen, carries away waste, helps detoxify the kidneys and liver, dissolves vitamins and minerals and cushions the body from injury by lubricating joints.

The human body is composed of 25 percent solid matter (the solute) and 75 percent water (the solvent). The average body contains 40 to 50 quarts of water. Your blood is 82 percent water, muscles are 75 percent water, the brain is 75 percent water and bone is 22 percent water.

Women have a tendency not to drink water for fear of constant trips to the bathroom or bloating. However, it is not the water that causes bloating but rather the excess salts and carbohydrates consumed that hold water in the body.

By the time you feel thirsty, you are probably already dehydrated. When you wake up in the morning, you have lost 10 to 12 glasses of water from the day before. You do not have to see perspiration to be losing a great deal of water. Simply by talking and breathing you are losing water.

Mild Dehydration-The Symptoms:

- Headache
- Dizziness
- Lethargy
- Mental fuzziness
- Loss of appetite
- Physical impairment

Dehydration can slow down your metabolism by 3%. If you are fighting a disease, have a cold or fever, are at a high altitude, on an airplane, are physically active, or if the weather is hot or humid you will need more water. Water is the body's air-conditioning system. When you become too warm, the loss of water through the pores of the skin, sweat glands and lungs prevents the body from building up too much internal heat.

Try to begin each day with 3 eight-ounce glasses of water and the same amount before each meal. Water is better and more easily consumed at room temperature. The average American consumes only half the recommended amount of water each day and an equal amount of dehydrating beverages which include any drink with caffeine or alcohol.

For every dehydrating drink, an additional glass of water is needed. When you become dehydrated, your body and brain become sluggish, your blood thickens and your heart is forced to work overtime.

Water is essential to life!

NOTE: For more information on water, I suggest that you read the wonderful book: *Your Body's Many Cries for Water* by Dr. F. Batmanghelidj.

- According to two of the world's leading experts, Richard Doll and Richard Peto of Oxford University, as many as 70 percent of all cancers may be related to diet. This is one statistic that jumped off the page for me. Although nutritional choices cannot change our genetic make-up, they can affect the personality of our genes by promoting healing and inhibiting cancer cells.

- "Certified Organic" means an authorized agency certified that the product was grown or raised without pesticides. If meat or poultry or dairy, that animal ate a vegetarian diet, was allowed to walk around to find food and was not given antibiotics.

- Pesticides, herbicides, industrial waste, antibiotics and hormones as well as artificial sweeteners and colorings play a role in Cancer promotion.

- Inside most cans (including soda cans) are trace amounts of a chemical called bisphenol A (BPA) which several researchers say has been linked to a pre-cancerous condition in mice. BPA is also found in plastic bottles and containers.

- Green tea consumption in women with breast cancer has resulted in fewer positive lymph nodes, and decreased recurrence by blocking growth factors of tumor promoters.

- You can not efficiently digest food if you eat too quickly. In fact you can suffer from malnutrition. Chewing your food stimulates the release of saliva in your stomach and digestive enzymes.

Things to Consider Before You Eat or Drink

Vanilla milkshake (32oz.)   1,010 calories/28 grams fat
Large French fries   600 calories/30 grams fat
Bagel with cream cheese   540 calories/22 grams fat
Organic Sorbet (1/2 cup)   120 calories/00 gram fat
Fresh Fruit Cup (8 oz.)   90 calories/01 gram fat

The EPA's list of the most commonly contaminated foods:

- Strawberries (the most heavily sprayed food on the market)
- Green and red bell peppers
- Spinach (tied)
- Cherries from the USA
- Peaches
- Cantaloupe from Mexico
- Celery
- Apples
- Green beans
- Grapes from Chile
- Cucumbers

The EPA's list of least commonly contaminated foods:

- Avocados (safest commercial food on the market)
- Corn
- Onions
- Sweet Potatoes
- Cauliflower
- Brussels sprouts
- Grapes USA
- Bananas
- Plums
- Scallion (green onions)
- Watermelon
- Broccoli

Increasingly, research suggests that getting the right amount of essential fatty acids is as important as getting your daily vitamins. EFAs are necessary to support a variety of cellular processes. They maintain cell walls and membranes, produce energy and hormones and help with normal brain, nerve and eye functions. They also aid in fighting off numerous health concerns such as elevated triglyceride and cholesterol levels, high blood pressure, rheumatoid arthritis, mental disorders, menstrual and menopausal symptoms, diabetic neuropathy, psoriasis and cancer.

Noted researcher Hugh Sinclair's theory linking fats and disease published in The Lancet, cites imbalances in fat metabolism as the underlying cause behind a number of diseases worldwide. Our modern diet, loaded with processed foods and hydrogenated fats or trans fats, is practically void of EFA's and is therefore the primary culprit.

Not consuming any fat at all is not healthy as it promotes hair loss and thinning, dryness of the skin and hair, eczema, joint problems, inflammations, PMS, depression and other mental disorders.

There are four EFAs that are essential to total body health.

ALA
Alpha linolenic acid, found in flaxseed. ALA has been shown to help the body in cancer prevention, protecting against heart disease and enhancing immune functions. Research has shown that 2 tablespoons of flaxseed daily slowed down tumor growth in breast cancer patients. The benefits of flax come from the high-lignan content of the flaxseed. You can purchase high-lignan flax seed oil from your health food store or grocer. Lignans are made up of cancer-fighting phytonutrients — antioxidants which normalize estrogen metabolism. You may also use it as a substitute for olive

oil, over vegetables and in the place of butter, but you can not cook with it. Flaxseed oil will dissipate if brought to high temperatures and you must keep it refrigerated.

GLA

Gamma linolenic acid is know for its effectiveness in fighting the effects of PMS, arthritis, cramping, headaches, irritability, burns, and skin enhancement. GLA may be synthesized from the raw material linoleic acid, found in vegetable oils, but disruptions caused by dietary factors prevent proper conversion. If you consume sugar, alcohol, and trans fats and lack minerals and vitamins in your diet you prevent the transformation of GLA. The richest sources of GLA are in borage oil, black current seed and evening primrose oil.

EPA and DHA

Omega-3s EPA and DHA have shown great promise in healing a variety of conditions such as high blood triglycerides, irregular heart beat, Crohn's disease, multiple sclerosis, lupus, cancer and hypertension. In January 2001, a landmark study was published in the Journal of the American Medical Association. The study discussed diets of 80,000 female nurses over a 14-year period and found that the risk of stroke due to blood clotting can be reduced by almost 50% by eating fish two to four times per week. Salmon is one of the best sources of omega-3s. It is recommended to eat at least two 3.oz servings of fatty fish per week. Sardines and mackerel are also good sources.

The bottom line: Getting all of your EFAs from food may not be easy for many, therefore it is important to consider taking EFAs as part of your basic supplementation program along with your multivitamins and minerals.

My childhood was rich with vegetables as I spent many days with my Grandmother Rosaria in what I called her "secret garden".

Carrots
In the last few years the world has come to know carrots and their healing effects when juiced. In North America and Europe alone there are more than 100 varieties. Not all carrots are only about beta-carotene, Vitamin A, fiber and their orange color. Have you ever savored one that is bright red, purple, yellow or white? When juicing carrots look for large Organic California juicing carrots as they are usually much sweeter than those grown in other parts of the country because of the high trace mineral content of the soil. Peeling your carrots before juicing will eliminate bacteria that may be present in the cracks or blemishes. Carrot juice reduces blood cholesterol, relieves constipation and other colon disorders, supports skin and tissue health, boosts the immune system, prevents heart and circulatory diseases and studies show that the beta-carotene in carrot juice helps to inhibit cancer cells and helps turn bad cells into good cells.

Beets and Beet Greens
Beets are very cleansing to the body and help to build red blood cells, protect against anemia, stimulate digestions, eliminate buildup of acid materials in the bowels, reduce cholesterol, aid the lymphatic system, protect the liver and gallbladder, cleanse the kidney and inhibit cancer cells. Beets are such powerful cleansers that it is best to use only a couple of ounces at one time and always combine with another juice. The greens or leaf hold the most nutrients and taste good when combined with carrots.

Raw Spinach
A rich source of Vitamins A and E as well as a source of iron. Spinach is also high in useable protein but should not be juiced alone.

Celery

When juicing celery, cut into half-inch pieces to prevent the strings from wrapping around the blade, which causes the motor in your juicer to overheat. Celery juice helps to alkalinize the bloodstream, purify the blood, improve digestion, aid kidney and liver functions, enhance the activity of white blood cells, halt fermentation and inhibit cancer cells. Celery is loaded with organic sodium, known as the element of youth and contains calcium, magnesium, potassium, Vitamin C and A.

Cabbage

Cabbage is part of the vegetable family known as cruciferous and contains more known anticancer properties than any other grouping. Included in this family are broccoli, Brussels sprouts, cauliflower, watercress, horseradish, kale, kohlrabi (turnip cabbage), mustard greens, radish, rutabaga and turnip.

Let's get started!

Purchase Organic fruits and vegetables to avoid poisonous chemicals found in pesticides.

Soak your produce for 15 minutes in a sink of water containing a cup of hydrogen peroxide. This will help remove parasites, bacteria and any chemical residues from the skin. This is especially important if not using organic produce.

When making juice of fruits and veggies, add 4 ounces of filtered or distilled water to 4 ounces of juice. Too much natural sugar from the juice can be hard on the pancreas.

Combining Fruits and Vegetables

The only fruits you can juice together with vegetables are apples and lemons, otherwise fruits and vegetables should never be mixed.

Apples
Any variety of apple will work to alkanize the blood, clean the bladder, ward off intestinal infections, reduce inflammation of the colon, reduce blood pressure, detoxify heavy metals from the system, and inhibit cancer cells.

Lemons
Lemon juice will add flavor and also contains cleansing properties which are good for the liver and gallbladder.

Facts About Juicing

Juices will lose most of their enzymes within about 30 minutes if exposed to the air. Drink immediately or store in a vacuum-sealed thermos. They will keep for about 8 hours in an air tight container.

A 72-hour juice fast will jump start your metabolism, help to purge toxins from your body, and allow healing and cleansing to take place. It is simple: the body works very hard to break down all that we consume. If we are only taking in juice the body has an opportunity to heal itself and dump toxic waste into the bloodstream that may have accumulated for years. These toxic wastes can then be purged from the body through any of the four pathways — the skin, lungs, kidneys and bowels. The bowels are the main passage. Enemas are used to help the toxic waste leave the body and not be reabsorbed through the colon wall. For more information on juice fasts and the use of enemas, please consult your homeopathic or naturopathic doctor.

The body is very resilient and has the ability to regenerate itself with a juice fast. Fasting helps the body to heal itself of more than we can imagine. Some benefits include energy, clearer skin, improved sleep, weight loss, reduction of allergies, heightened senses, change in eating habits and deeper relaxation.

The Scoop on Juicing Machines

Centrifugal Juicers
These have spinning baskets that rotate at a very high rate of speed (usually 5,000 to 6,000 revolutions per minute), shredding food and flinging juice through the air causing oxidation to take place. This shredding action is not very effective in breaking open the cells to extract the nutrients from the pulp.

Masticating Juicers
These operate at much lower speeds and have the capability to be used as grinders for nuts, seeds, grains and dried fruit. These juicers can also make nut butters, breads, and frozen banana ice cream. These juicers include:

- The Champion Juicer   **Approximate Cost $300**

This juicer has hundreds of teeth that revolve at 1725 revolutions per minute. After this juicer has shredded the carrots, it presses the pulp against a stainless steel screen forcing out more nutrients. It will yield about the same amount of juice as the centrifugal juicers but tests show that this machine will yield three to four times more nutrients. This is a good low-end juicer.

- The Green Star Juicer   **Approximate Cost $500**

This is the only juicer that does not use knife blades to extract juice. Rather it uses twin gears to revolve at only 110rpm. The twin gears draw the food down and press out the juice in an airtight chamber, without pumping oxygen into the juice. Laboratory reports show that it yields approximately 10 more ounces of juice from a 5 pound bag of carrots then the centrifugal or Champion juicer while doubling the nutrients of the Champion.

- The Norwalk Press Juicer **Approximate Cost $ 2,000**

This has large, heavy-duty knife blades that force pulp and juice through a fine strainer. The shredded pulp and juice then drops into a cloth bag. The bag is then placed onto a hydraulic press (part of the same juicer) and the bag of shredded pulp is pressed under great pressure. This juicer yields about 16 ounces more than the Champion Juicer and 6 ounces more than the Green Star Juicer. This is a rather costly investment as the Champion and Green Star will provide adequate nutrients.

www.diamondorganics.com
Since 1990, the nation's premiere source of farm-fresh organic food with guaranteed overnight home delivery to most destinations.

www.christinacooks.com
Christina Pirello, a leukemia survivor and star of Christina Cooks Naturally, shares her love for cooking naturally and the healing of her own body.

www.wholefoods.com
The world's leading natural and organic foods supermarket.

www.hacres.com
Good site to order Barley Max, Fibercleanse and other supplements to help cleanse and boost the immune system. One of my favorite recipe books—*"Recipes for Life from God's Garden,"* by Rhonda J. Malkmus—is available here.

www.TKfitness.com
Name-brand supplements at wholesale prices, one of the best in the U.S.

www.johnmasters.com
This lovely soothing salon is a must-see if in NYC. John Masters has been in the hair care business for over 25 years, since he began creating organic hair products from his home.

www.realgoods.com
Alternative products to create a healthy environment.

www.docharrison.com
Natural, safe products to care for your teeth and gums.

Nutritious and delicious, this is my personal recipe for a complete meal which includes a combination of protein, carbohydrates and good fat.

In your blender:

4-6 oz.	Organic Rice or Almond Milk
20-30 Grams	Vegan Brown Rice Protein
1 tbsp.	High-Lignan Flax Seed Oil
1 tbsp.	Organic honey

Add your favorite ORGANIC fruit such as strawberries, peaches, blueberries, banana, pineapple, etc.
Clean, cut and freeze fruit in advance to make for a thicker drink.
Add crushed ice from filtered water.
*Add other vitamins or herbs as needed.
Blend at a high speed.

Enjoy!   Glass size: 8oz.   Calories: 350

NOTE: Taking fiber on an empty stomach 30 minutes before eating will help your digestion. I take Renew Life Organic Triple Fiber with Flax Seed, Oat Bran & Acacia.

I also take a certified organic whole-food concentrate made from the juice of young barley grass and alfalfa called BarleyMax. This is similar to having a shot of wheat grass from your local juice bar. Take on an empty stomach 20 minutes before eating.
See www.hacres.com to order this product.

- Organically grown fruits and vegetables including cruciferous vegetables such as broccoli, cauliflower, kale, bok choy, and Brussels sprouts

- Organic olive oil

- Fresh organic garlic

- Organic whole grains: brown rice, quinoa, amaranth and barley

- Organic high-lignan flaxseed oil or flaxseeds (you will need a grinder)

- Organic green tea

- Organic spices: oregano, basil, turmeric, rosemary

- Wakame or mekabu seaweed

- Organic Brazil nuts, almonds, cashews

- Organic dried fruits: apricots, mangos, apples, pineapple

- Non-toxic laundry detergent, household cleaning supplies and personal-care items

This is my personal plan for breast prevention and maintenance. **Please speak with your nutritionist or doctor before making changes to your diet.**

1. Eat plenty of organic fruits, vegetables and whole grains

Plant foods contain dozen of vitamins and minerals that all help to protect you against cancer.

2. Go for the Good Fats

See my chapter: Healthy Fats.

3. Drink Green Tea

Rich in antioxidants, it promotes good health. Start with 1-2 cups per day and work up to 4-5 cups. I purchase all of my teas from www.stashtea.com.

4. Include Flax Seed

You will need to grind these seeds to add them to smoothies and apple juice or sprinkle them on top of fruit, cereal or salads.

5. Sleep from 9PM to 6AM

These are the best hours to boost levels of protective cancer hormones, especially melatonin. Sleep is the time when your cells can heal.

6. Use Supplements that Fight Cancer

Turmeric – A good anti-cancer spice which helps the body neutralize environmental toxins and shut off the blood supply to tumors. It also enhances live enzymes and acts as an anti-inflammatory.

Selenium – A mineral that helps the body inhibit the formation of tumors and may slow their growth.

CoQ10 – Low levels of this enzyme have been found in breast cancer patients therefore supplementing may reduce risk.

7. Take Charge

Obtain copies of all of your test results and start a binder in chronological order. The nurse in my doctor's was very helpful in teaching me how to read the tests. Ask your doctor to make a note to have all test results mailed to you.

8. Be Informed

Education is the key. Continue to do research and be up on the latest information.

9. Let Family and Friends Help

Chances are that if you have just been diagnosed with breast cancer, your family and friends are feeling helpless. Put them to work to help you. Taking a friend or family member along to doctors' visits or tests will make for good company, and you get hugs too!

10. Be a Good Patient.

Develop a good relationship with your doctors and have an open and direct dialogue with them. Find doctors who have compassion, and will take time to answer your questions. You need to trust the doctors you have entrusted with your care. Most of all be honest with your doctor and expect the same.

11. Eat Smart

Nutrition is the secret to good health.

12. Don't Smoke

This is the leading cause of death in North America and a risk factor for breast cancer.

13. Avoid Alcohol

Alcohol dehydrates your body. Please use in moderation.

14. Exercise

Get moving for at least 30 minutes daily to improve your body, bones, mind and reduce stress. Being fit helps you look and feel your best!

15. Be Happy

A healthy, positive outlook will bring healing to your body and mind. Seek out what works best for you and practice it every day.

REFERENCES

- All About Breast Cancer Overview www.cancer.org

- National Women's Health Resource Center Web Site

- Fasting as a Way of Life, Alan Cott, M.D.

- Your Body's Cry For Water, F. Batmanghelidj, M.D.

- Dr. Merrick I. Ross, M.D., F.A.C.S

PERSONAL NOTES

PERSONAL NOTES